CANCER

CAUSES, PREVENTION & TREATMENT

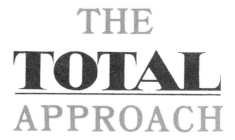

THE
TOTAL
APPROACH

A research paper delivered at the Ninth Annual
CANCER Convention of the International Association
of Cancer Victims and Friends.

by PAAVO O. AIROLA, N.D., Ph.D.

HEALTH PLUS, PUBLISHERS
P. O. BOX 22001, PHOENIX, ARIZONA 85028

FIRST PRINTING, AUGUST, 1972
SECOND PRINTING, MAY, 1973
THIRD PRINTING, APRIL, 1974
FOURTH PRINTING, MARCH, 1975
FIFTH PRINTING, FEBRUARY, 1976
SIXTH PRINTING, MARCH, 1977
SEVENTH PRINTING, JANUARY, 1978
EIGHTH PRINTING, DECEMBER, 1978
NINTH PRINTING, DECEMBER, 1979
TENTH PRINTING, JANUARY, 1981
ELEVENTH PRINTING, OCTOBER, 1982
TWELFTH PRINTING, NOVEMBER, 1983

Printed in the U.S.A.

CANCER
CAUSES, PREVENTION AND TREATMENT
The TOTAL Approach

IMPORTANT NOTES

From the Publisher:

The information in this book is presented for educational purposes only; it is not intended as diagnosing or prescribing. In the event the reader uses the information to solve his own health problems, he is prescribing for himself, which is his constitutional right, but the author and the publisher assume no responsibility.

We strongly advise that when cancer is suspected, under no circumstances should home remedies, nutritional or any other kind, be tried. Instead, a reliable doctor, preferably biologically and nutritionally oriented, should be consulted immediately, and the patient should abide by the doctor's advice regarding most suitable therapies, including the therapies presented in this book.

From the Author:

I wish to stress the fact that I do not own nor do I have any financial or economic interest in any of the spas and clinics mentioned in this book. Likewise, I do not sell any of the vitamins, supplements or other products mentioned or recommended in the book. I do not own health food stores and I am not connected with any vitamin or food supplement manufacturing or retailing industry. The sole reason for writing this book is to help the reader by giving him vital information which I uncovered through years of study and research.

PAAVO O. AIROLA

TABLE OF CONTENTS

INTRODUCTION

First I want to make it perfectly clear* that I do **not** offer a **cure for cancer.** I only report how cancer is successfully treated in several of the biological clinics in Europe, particularly in Germany, but also in Denmark, Sweden and Switzerland.

There are several hundred so-called biological clinics in Europe, most of them directed by medical doctors, where drugless, biological medicine is practiced. In my book, **THERE IS A CURE FOR ARTHRITIS,** I list over a dozen such clinics with the complete addresses and names of the doctors. The most prominent cancer specialists in Germany using biological therapies in the treatment of cancer are Dr. Josef Issels, Prof. Werner Zabel, Dr. Ernst Mayer, Dr. Hans Nieper, Prof. Werner Kollath and Prof. Lampert. But there are over 4,000 medical doctors in Germany, members of the Association of Naturopathic (Biological) Doctors, who apply biological therapies in the treatment of most diseases, including cancer.

All my statements made in regard to the causes of cancer, and to effective nutritional and other biological methods of approaching the cancer treatment, are well documented — see the references.

Again, I do not offer a new or any other kind of cure for cancer — I report only what various cancer researchers have found and how cancer is successfully treated in European biological clinics. In this country all harmless, unorthodox treatments of cancer are outlawed leaving only surgery, radiation or chemotherapy. I feel that the millions of people who suffer from cancer are entitled to know the truth.

*Mainly to protect myself against persecution by over-zealous government agencies who, in the name of protecting the public, mercilessly attack anyone who not only dares to advise but even to report on unorthodox cancer therapies.

The basic causes of cancer, as well as the effective methods of prevention, control and treatment of cancer, have been known for a long time. It is the responsibility of all sincere and dedicated men to make this knowledge available so it can be applied to the benefit of all those who suffer, or will suffer, from this dreadful disease of civilization — cancer.

WHAT CAUSES CANCER

A few days ago I was discussing the cancer question with some of my new friends. They emphasized the hopelessness of the situation, mentioning the fact that although this dreadful disease — cancer — kills millions of people, no one really knows what causes cancer, in which case there is no hope in sight for the speedy discovery of a cure or remedy for this catastrophic situation. They mentioned the fact that the President of the United States, Richard Nixon, is extremely concerned with the increasing incidence of cancer and that the Congress of the United States, in addition to billions already spent, has allocated 1.6 billion dollars of our tax money to "accelerate research aimed at finding the cause and cure of cancer."

I said to my friends:

"What a waste of money! If President Nixon and the governmental health authorities really want to find out what causes cancer and how to eliminate it, all they have to do is to spend an 8 cent stamp writing a letter to me — I can tell them **exactly** what the real causes of cancer are and how cancer can be wiped out completely. And I will give them this valuable information free — it won't cost the taxpayers a penny, and they can save billions of dollars and millions of lives!"

As you can imagine, my new friends looked at me with sympathetic and pitying smiles, as if saying: "Brother, we've heard that you were a nut and a crackpot — but we never dreamed that you were that far out!" And then came the line that most of you, I am sure, have heard before:

"Dr. Airola, if you really knew the cause and the cure of cancer, you wouldn't be sitting here right now in this middle class home and driving a Maverick. You would be not only one of the most famous people in the world, but also one of the wealthiest!"

The average layman, doctor, or scientist in this country is still convinced that the cause of cancer is unknown. Billions of dollars are spent on so-called research aimed mainly at trying to find a virus that causes cancer.

Yet, I dare to proclaim to you and to the whole world that I know exactly what causes cancer — and in the next half an hour you will agree, I am sure, that my claims are based on 100% proven scientific facts.

SCIENTIFICALLY AND EMPIRICALLY PROVEN CAUSES OF CANCER

I will enumerate some of the proven causes of cancer — causes that are well known to you and to every cancer researcher in the world.

1. EXCESSIVE SMOKING

It has been established beyond the shadow of a doubt by world-wide research and endorsed by the U.S. Surgeon General, that excessive smoking causes cancer in the lungs, stomach, respiratory organs, lips and mouth.[1]

2. SUN

It has been established conclusively by numerous studies that excessive and continuous exposure to the sun's ultraviolet rays can cause cancer of the skin in some people. Rimless eyeglasses, which concentrate the sun's reflections, are particularly dangerous and are responsible for many cases of skin cancer on the face.[2,3]

3. MECHANICAL, PHYSICAL AND CHEMICAL IRRITATION

Prolonged physical irritation of the skin or mucous membranes can cause cancer. Classic examples: smoker's pipe or "tailor's needle" can cause cancer of the lips. Prolonged irritation by ill-fitted dentures can cause cancer of the tongue or gums. Excessive and continued drinking of very hot beverages may cause cancer of the throat and/or stomach. Prolonged irritation of the skin by chemicals or drugs may cause skin cancer. Prolonged irritation of warts, pimples or slow-healing sores may result in malignant tumors.[3]

These common causes of cancer by mechanical, physical or chemical irritation have been known for centuries.

4. DES or DIETHYLSTILBESTROL

A recent report by the FDA, based on extensive research from the U.S. and many other countries, shows that diethylstilbestrol is definitely a causative factor in cancer of the uterus, breast and other reporductive organs.[4,5] Diethylstilbestrol is an artificial sex hormone widely used in food production. It has been established that 85% of all meat in the United States contains dangerous residues of stilbestrol. This is the main reason why 15 countries around the world now refuse to import American meat.

By the way, cancer is not the only thing stilbestrol causes. It also destroys both fertility and sexual libido in men. It is a well known secret that during the last two decades there was a dramatic decrease in virility of American men who are traditionally heavy meat eaters. Stilbestrol, this artificial female sex hormone, is feminizing our men, while it speeds up sexual maturity in young girls. In recent years, the average age of sexual maturity in young girls has dropped from sixteen to twelve or thirteen years.[6]

Do you know that 21 nations around the world have a total ban on the use of stilbestrol in food production or food processing, while the FDA still permits its wide use in this country?

5. CYCLAMATES

The FDA has recently banned the artificial sweetener, **cyclamate**, which has been widely used for decades in food processing and bottled drinks. It has been established in animal studies that cyclamates can cause cancer in the stomach and in other digestive organs. As a direct result of years of use of cyclamates, some doctors express the fear that cancer will continue to develop in the digestive organs for decades to come.[7]

6. SACCHARIN

Cyclamates are not the only artificial sweetener that can cause cancer. There is another artificial sweetener that was discovered almost 100 years ago and has been widely used since then — saccharin. As recently as February of this year, the FDA ordered saccharin removed from its G R A S list. (GRAS means Generally Recognized As Safe). Reliable animal tests conducted by a University of Wisconsin research team showed that saccharin causes cancer in the bladder and uterus. Of course, the removal of saccharin from the G R A S list does not mean that it is banned from sale or use. In the United States over five million pounds of saccharin is used by the food industry each year.

7. NITROSAMINES

It has been scientifically proven in actual studies that nitrosamines cause cancer of the liver, stomach, brain, bladder, kidneys and several other organs. Nitrosamines are produced in the body from nitrites and nitrates, chemical preservatives and color enhancers commonly used today, especially in all processed meat products. Dr. William Lijinski, famous research scientist from the Cancer Research Center of the University of Nebraska, says: "Nitrosamines are perfect carcinogens" — they can cause cancer anywhere in the body.

If you ate any meat today, more likely than not carcinogenic nitrosamines are building up in your body right now. Nitrates and nitrites can also enter the body in drinking water, most of which is contaminated by argicultural nitrate-containing chemical fertilizers.

8. HEXACHLOROPHENE

By a recent FDA action, hexachlorophene was indicted as a possible carcinogen. Hexachlorophene causes brain damage and cancer in the brain. It is used widely in maternal and other wards of hospitals and is also present in many cosmetics, soaps, deodorants and other toilet articles.

9. SMOG

Ozone, carbon monoxide, nitrogen dioxide and other photochemical pollutants in common smog have been indicted by many researchers as definite carcinogens.[8] Smog now covers most of this country and none of us can escape the carcinogenic effects of it. Carcinogenic chemicals present in smog cause many health disorders, including cancer, particularly in the lungs and other respiratory organs.

10. COAL TAR DYES

Many artificial coloring substances produced from coal tar are shown to be highly carcinogenic; yet they are still allowed to be used in foods, soft drinks, cosmetics, medicines, etc.[9]

11. STRONTIUM 90

Strontium 90 is a radioactive substance that is now present almost everywhere on this globe as a result of radioactive fallout from atomic tests and bomb explosions. It finds its way into the human body through food, particularly milk. The famous Russian scientist, Dr. A. V. Topchiev, said recently: "Much of the rising incidence of leukemia and sarcoma of the bone is caused by strontium 90."[10]

12. IODINE 131

In addition to strontium 90, another radioactive chemical, called iodine 131, which also comes from atomic fallout, is proven carcinogen.[11]   It has been definitely established that radioactive iodine causes cancer of the thyroid gland. Iodine 131 is present in large amounts in our environment and food, mostly in milk — and is, therefore, of particular danger to children.

13

Please keep in mind that radioactive iodine and strontium 90 fallout is not limited to commercial farming — they fall on and contaminate organic farms and gardens as well.

In Hiroshima, those who survived lethal doses of atomic fallout, developed leukemia after about 5 years, and cancer after 20 years. This proves that it may take several decades after exposure to carcinogens before cancer developes to a diagnosable stage.

13. EXCESSIVE X-RAYS

It has been scientifically proven that not only excessive x-rays, but even the kind that are used prophylactically or diagnostically by doctors, dentists and chiropractors, can cause cancer and leukemia. Leukemia in children in later years is often caused by prenatal abdominal x-rays received by the mother during pregnancy.[12]

14. CADMIUM

Although beneficial in minute amounts, the trace element, **cadmium**, is extremely toxic in larger amounts. It is present in increasing amounts in our environment mostly from automobiles, phosphate fertilizers and various industries. It pollutes the soil and the water, and is taken up by plants, particularly by cereal grains. By the way, according to Dr. Lars Friberg, of Sweden, wheat takes up 10 times as much cadmium as rice. It is concentrated in animal livers, which makes liver a very dangerous food, indeed. Shellfish also concentrate cadmium to dangerous levels.

Cadmium can cause many serious health disorders, such as high blood pressure, heart disease, iron-deficiency anemia, emphysema, chronic bronchitis, lung fibrosis, kidney damage — and cancer.[13]

15. DRUGS AND ENVIRONMENTAL CHEMICALS

We are living in an era of unprecedented chemical assault from every direction. Our air, our water, and our food contains thousands of man-made toxic chemicals, most of them potential carcinogens. According to Dr. Alfred Taylor, of the

Biology Institute of the University of Texas, even sodium fluoride in fluoridated water, which almost one half of all Americans are now forced to drink, is linked to cancer growth.[14]   Many commonly used drugs are considered by many researchers to be possible carcinogens. [15, 16]

Also, many widely used pesticides are definite carcinogens.[17]   Animal studies commissioned by HEW and conducted by Bionetics Research Laboratories of Bethesda, Maryland, showed that more than half of all mice given oral doses of DDT developed tumors. In spite of mounting evidence that DDT is a proven carcinogen, and in spite of the fact that many countries in Europe had banned DDT completely, DDT is still permitted and widely used on food crops in the United States, although the public is given an impression that it is already banned. Here in California it is still permitted on alfalfa seed crops, onions, citrus fruit, and peppers.[18]

16. SALT

What? Common salt a carcinogen? Yes, even this common chemical, sodium chloride, if used in excessive amounts, can cause cancer.[19]   World Health Organization (WHO), an auxiliary of the United Nations, reported from Japan that it has been statistically demonstrated that the frequency of cancer of the stomach in Japan is definitely related to the quantity of salt consumed by the natives. The more salt in the diet — the more stomach cancer. [20]

17. RANCID FOODS AND OILS

Modern food processing and marketing methods mean progress to some. To me, they are something else. With the emphasis on long shelf-life, many foods are stale and rancid before they are consumed. This is particularly true in regard to natural, unprocessed, so-called health foods. Such widely used health foods as wheat germ, wheat germ oil, sunflower seeds, sesame seeds and whole wheat flour are marvelous health-building "wonder" foods — **if eaten absolutely fresh!** It is, however, virtually impossible to obtain them fresh.

Natural, unprocessed foods are extremely perishable. Wheat germ turns rancid one week after it is made (it is always much older than that when delivered to the stores). Rancid foods are extremely dangerous. Not only are the vitamins, such as vitamine E, A and F, for which we eat many of these foods, totally destroyed in rancid foods, but, during the process of becoming rancid, extremely harmful chemical substances, such as peroxides and others, are formed. These, by virtue of being strong chemical irritants, can cause cancer. This is acknowledged by the foremost authority on rancid foods in the world, Dr. H. Anemueller, of Germany, and in animal studies made by Drs. Rownee and Barrett of the University of Pennsylvania.[21]

Also heated fats, particularly vegetable fats heated to a high temperature, become carcinogenic.[22,23]

18. HIGH ANIMAL PROTEIN DIET

Dr. Josef Issels, perhaps the foremost cancer specialist in the world and director of his world famous cancer clinic, says:

"Excessive eating of meat and other cholesterol-rich foods not only contributes to atherosclerosis and consequent impaired blood circulation and diminished oxygenation of cells, but also increases the risk of tumor development. Animal as well as human studies show that limiting the use of meat and animal fats, including butter, will diminish the risk of cancer.[24, 25]

Overconsumption of protein not only causes deficiencies of vitamin B_6, B_3 and magnesium, but also a chronic pancreatic enzyme deficiency, considered to be one of the main causes of cancer in the countries with high protein consumption.[26] It can be statistically demonstrated that the countries with high animal protein consumption have a greater incidence of cancer. And, contrariwise, countries where the traditional diet is low in animal protein — even low in any kind of protein — have little or no cancer at all. The people of Hunza are just one example where the diet is extremely low in protein, especially animal protein. Many others could be mentioned, like the Yucatan Indians or the Todas in East India, where people eat only a fraction of the typical American protein intake and where cancer is unknown. Americans eat more protein than any other country in the world. We also lead the world in cancer statistics. Most leading cancer researchers and nutritionally-oriented doctors, such as Dr. Max Gerson, Dr. Josef Issels, Dr. Werner Zabel, Dr. William Kelley, Dr. Ernst Krebs, Dr. Werner Kollath and Dr. Alan H. Nittler, to name a few, are convinced that overindulgence in protein and the body's inability to properly digest and utilize it is one of the prime causes of cancer.

19. OVEREATING

Almost everyone agrees that obesity is one of the main causes of most so-called diseases of civilization, or the degenerative diseases: arthritis, diabetes, heart disease — and cancer. Metropolitan Life statistics show that the prevalence of these diseases among the overweight is far greater than among those of normal weight. According to Dr. Issels, animal studies show that the animals allowed to eat as much as they wished had 5.3 times more spontaneous cancer tumors than those animals who fasted every second day.[24, 27] The hunger years during and immediately after both World Wars resulted in a virtual disappearance of cancer, as well as of most other diseases of civilization. When food rationing was abandoned, cancer statistics soared rapidly back to a pre-war level. Even such a conservative organization as the National Cancer Institute acknowledges the relationship between overeating and cancer. Their official publication, "The Challenge of Cancer." states, "There is statistical evidence from various insurance companies that overweight persons have a distinctly greater tendency for developing cancer."[28]

20. ABNORMAL REPRODUCTIVE AND SEXUAL PATTERNS

It has been established that increasingly prevalent cancer of the prostate gland in men is often caused by such unnatural practices as irregularity of or undue abstinence from sexual gratification. As our society abandons the old sexual, marital and maternal traditions, cancer in the reproductive organs becomes more and more prevalent. Mothers who do not breast feed their offspring run a greater risk of breast cancer. Such practices as heavy petting which leads to a high degree of sexual excitation without the natural conclusion, the practice of withdrawal or deliberate prolongation of the sex act — all these can contribute to prostate disorders and increase the risk of prostate cancer.[6]

21. NUTRITIONAL DEFICIENCIES

According to recent statistics from the U.S. Department of Agriculture and the U.S. Department of Health, Education and Welfare, about 50% — **one half!** — of all Americans suffer from various degrees of malnutrition and nutritional deficiences. It has been shown in more than a hundred studies from around the world that almost any serious nutritional deficiency of one or more vitamins, minerals or other nutritive substances can lower the resistances to spontaneous cancer and increase the risk of contracting the disease. For example:

- Even a mild deficiency of choline will produce cancer of the liver.[29, 30]
- Vitamin E deficiency increases the risk of contracting cancer[31] and leukemia.[32]
- An iodine deficient diet has resulted in cancer, mostly of the thyroid gland.[33]
- Deficiencies of various B-vitamins result in liver damage which leads to malignancies.[16, 34]
- Serious deficiency of the mineral zinc may lead to cancer of the prostate.[35]
- Vitamin A deficiency breaks down the body's defenses against most carcinogens and leads to tumor development[36]

- Magnesium deficiency is also linked to cancer development, as shown in studies conducted at the University of Montreal and in Egypt.[37]

And so on. Since nutritional deficiencies are so wide-spread in this country, they must constitute a large causative factor in cancer development.

22. SEVERE EMOTIONAL STRESS

Finally, more and more, valid research tends to indicate that personality traits play an important part in cancer development. Dr. Helen Flanders Dunbar claims "that only certain types of people succumb to cancer."[38]   Popular health pioneer, J.I. Rodale, claimed that "happy people don't get cancer." Recent studies by such researchers as Dr. L. LeShan, of the Institute of Applied Biology at New York University, Dr. Arthur Schmale, Jr. and Dr. Howard Iker of the University of Rochester Medical Center, and Dr. William Greene, Jr. of the University of Rochester Medical Center, all came up with similar findings: Certain types of people, people with a lowered ability to deal with severe emotional conflicts and stresses, people with uncontrolled anxieties and worries, those with traumatic emotional experiences or losses, those with feelings of loneliness, inadequacy, hopelessness and desperation, people who could be classified generally as hopeless or unhappy — these types of people are more predisposed to to succumb to cancer. Investigators emphasize that although such a negative state of mind may not cause cancer in and of itself, it increases the biochemical vulnerability and sets the stage for cancer growth.[39]

Now, after enumerating all these 22 causes of cancer, (and I could name 22 more) all scientifically and empirically well-proven causes, wouldn't you agree with me that **we actually DO KNOW what causes cancer?!**

The primary and ultimate cause of cancer is lowered or broken down resistance of the body's own defense mechanism against the singular or combined physical, chemical,

19

emotional and environmental stresses that I've just enumerated. The unprecedented chemical insult from the environment, air, water and food, dietary abuses and deficiencies, overindulgence, particularly in proteins, severe emotional stresses, faulty and health-destroying living habits — these prolonged stresses lower or break down the body's resistance against disease and pave the way for the development of cancer.

Why then, in spite of the fact that all these causes of cancer have been known for a long time, do we hear repeated statements that we still do not know what causes cancer, and why do the government and research institutions, paid with our tax money, spend billions of dollars trying to find the cause of cancer? Why?

It is an interesting question. And I have some interesting — and shocking — answers to it. However, I was asked by the officials of this Association to refrain from attacking certain vested interests or bringing politics or religion into the discussion — furthermore, I do not look well in stripes! But I will make a couple of statements:

1. Our American medical system is a profit-oriented professional monopolistic organization built on the principle: **the more sickness — the more profit.** Thus, the total elimination of disease, be it cancer or anything else, is contrary to the basic economic interests of our medical-drug-hospital industry complex.

2. Disease is a big business — an 80 billion-dollar-a-year business.

3. Cancer represents one of the biggest sources of income to the medical-drug-hospital industry.

Now you can form your own conclusions as to why billions of dollars are spent on the search for a non-existent virus as a cause of cancer, and why we are not getting anywhere in the battle against this dreadful disease.

HOW CANCER CAN BE ELIMINATED

But let's get back to where we finished regarding the causes of cancer.

Now that we agree that we actually **do know** the real causes of cancer — what is the next logical step? Simple: now that the basic causes of cancer are known, we can completely eliminate cancer from the American scene **BY ELIMINATING THE CAUSES OF CANCER.**

As we have seen, the basic causes of cancer are tied in with our environment, with our way of life, with our nutrition, with our living habits. By changing our living habits, by improving our nutrition, by eliminating all the known carcinogens from our environment, from our food, water and air, we can completely wipe out this disease of civilization. As Are Waerland, my teacher and friend, said: "We do not deal with diseases — only with mistakes in our way of living; eliminate the mistakes — and diseases will disappear of their own accord."[40]

When all the cancer-causing and cancer-inducing factors are eliminated from our lives, cancer will disappear and "will be no more", just as it is non-existent in Hunza. This is the only way the victory over cancer will ever be won. Stop smoking, stop polluting our air, stop devitalizing and destroying our food, stop poisoning air, water and soil with carcinogenic chemicals, stop the health-destroying high-protein fad, stop the mad race for more material prosperity and adopt a contented mental attitude, eat natural, unprocessed foods, breath pure air, drink pure water, live close to nature and do your daily quota of perspiring either by hard physical work or exercise — and you can forget about cancer! **Cancer will vanish forever — not because we cured it, but**

21

because we eliminated the causes for its existence.

More billions of dollars given to so-called cancer research will be nothing but a monumental loss of money. Only a radical change in our life pattern, a change from the **health-destroying** to the **health-building** life style, will turn the tide and help us conquer cancer.

Thus, the ultimate road to a total elimination of cancer is not in **finding a cure,** but in adopting massive cancer-preventive programs which would make cancer obsolete.

CAN CANCER BE CURED?

Now, I am sure, most of you agree with this prevention idea. But I am also sure that here in this audience there are hundreds of people who are already afflicted by this disease; and hundreds more have friends or relatives affected by it. The prevention approach is too late for them. They would like to know: **what can be done to help them?** Are there any alternatives to the surgery, radiation and chemotherapy that orthodox medicine offers them, alternatives that are safe, harmless and effective? Are there any new approaches in the nutritional and biological medical field that can help them and their friends?

Cancer has been successfully treated in some European biological clinics. Dr. Josef Issels' cancer clinic in Germany is particularly known in this field.[58] There were some excellent cancer clinics in the United States also, like Dr. Max Gerson's clinic, for example, but they are closed now, unfortunately. Harmless, effective — but unorthodox— therapies are not allowed to be employed in this supposedly free country. In Europe there is still a somewhat more tolerant attitude towards natural methods of cancer treatment. I will introduce you to some of these.

First, let me state that the European approach to cancer is a combined attack on all fronts, the total mobilization of all known anti-cancer factors. All measures and treatments know to help in detoxifying the body, stimulating the vital body organs and functions, improving glandular activity and increasing and strengthening the body's own healing forces, are employed simultaneously for maximum effect.

Americans are, generally speaking, a drug-oriented people. We are always looking for a single drug, a pill, that will cure or control the condition. This is also true in regard to cancer. Although drugs may be effective in controlling the symptoms, I am thoroughly convinced that no drug or pill will be found that will cure cancer, just as there is no drug in existence that will cure any disease. Disease — any disease, including cancer — can be cured only by the body's own healing mechanism. In fact, disease, as we know it, that is, the outward symptoms of disease, is nothing but the body's manifestation of its own defensive and remedial effort to correct the adverse condition and restore health. A tumor is nothing but the body's effort to isolate the affected cells in order to protect the rest of the organism, and extend life. Therefore, the effective cure for any disease can be accomplished only **from within**, by the body's own extensive healing mechanism. We are equipped with a marvelous healing system, more effective than any healing system devised by man. This built-in healing system is capable of correcting any condition of ill health if given the opportunity and proper conditions. Consequently, the first principle of biological medicine is to create conditions most conducive to self-healing, to support, stimulate and activate the body's own healing activity with all the known harmless and effective means.

The combined biological attack against cancer, the TOTAL approach, includes the following proven and effective supportive measures:

1. ARTIFICIALLY INDUCED FEVER

"Give me a chance to create fever and I will cure any disease," said the great ancient physician Parmenides. Many modern giants of biological medicine in Europe, such as the Nobel Prize winner, Dr. A. Lwoff,[41] famous German cancer specialist, Prof. Werner Zabel,[42] and the director of the most successful cancer clinic in the world, the Ringberg-Klinik, Dr. Josef Issels, use artificially induced fever in their battle against cancer.[42]

Dr. Werner Zabel told the following true story, which illustrates the cancer-preventive and cancer-healing effect of artificially induced fever:

Not far from Rome, Italy, there were huge swampy areas called the Pontine Swamps. These swamps were excellent breeding grounds for malaria mosquitoes, and the whole area was affected by malaria.

Then, by government action, the Pontine Swamps were drained and dried out. As a result malaria completely disappeared. But Italian medical researchers made a remarkable observation. While earlier the whole malaria-infected area was completely free from cancer, now, one generation later, it had the same prevalence of cancer as the rest of Italy. The scientists concluded that the frequent fever attacks common in malaria stimulated the body's own defenses so that cancer could not develop.

Fever has been too long a misunderstood and mistreated symptom. Most orthodox doctors try to combat and suppress fever. Actually fever is a constructive, health-promoting symptom, initiated and created by the body in its own effort to fight infections and other conditions of disease and to restore health. High temperature speeds up metabolism, inhibits the growth of invading virus or bacteria and accelerates the healing processes.

In folk medicine in various parts of the world fever has been used for centuries to heal disease. In the West Indies, natives afflicted with syphilis or cancer cured themselves by deliberately subjecting themselves to infection from such high fever diseases as malaria, typhus fever or typhoid fever.

Dr. A. Lwoff, famous French bacteriologist, has demonstrated in repeated scientific experiments that fever is indeed a "great medicine," and that if can help to cure many "incurable diseases". In biological clinics in Europe, artificially induced fever, mostly in the form of overheating baths, has been used successfully to treat such conditions as rheumatic diseases, skin disorders, insomnia, arthritis — and cancer. Dr. Josef Issels has said, "Artificially induced fever has the greatest potential in the treatment of many diseases, including cancer." Mark well that this remark is made by one of the leading cancer specialists in the world!

The usual method of inducing fever is the so-called Schlenz-bath.[43] The patient is totally immersed in a large bathtub filled with water between 100-102 degrees Farenheit. Only the nose and mouth are left free for breathing. In about half an hour, the body's temperature will gradually rise to match the temperature of the water.

Needless to say, treatment should be given by the nurse and should be well supervised. The temperature of the water and of the patient, and the patient's pulse, should be checked periodically. (Detailed instructions for administering the Schlenz-bath are given in my book, **Health Secrets From Europe.**[43]

2. THE ANTI-CANCER DIET

This may shock some orthodox cancer specialists in the United States, but according to the leading biological cancer specialists in Europe (Zabel, Issels, Kollath, Meyer, Lampert, Kuhl, Warburg, et al.) there is, indeed, such a thing as an anti-cancer diet — a diet that can help prevent cancer, as well as help the body to cure cancer.

In order to help the body prevent cancer, or to assist the body's healing activity when cancer is already developed, Dr. Issels advises the following anti-cancer diet:[24]

1. Diet must consist exclusively of bio-dynamically (organically) grown foods, which are free from carcinogenic chemi-

cals, such as toxic additives, insecticide residues, preservatives and other man-made chemicals.

2. Most foods must be eaten in their natural, raw state. The diet doesn't have to be 100% raw, although it should be at least 80% to 90% raw. Certain foods, such as soybeans, buckwheat, millet, rice and some dried beans, could be cooked.

3. Emphasis should be on raw vegetables, fruits, nuts, and sprouted seeds and grains. The best nuts are almonds, walnuts and filberts. Peanuts should be avoided by cancer patients. Although peanuts are excellent food, they are often infected by a yellow fungus which is carcinogenic. The best anti-cancer grains are: millet, buckwheat, brown rice and barley.

4. Anti-cancer diet should include generous amounts of fermented (lactic acid) foods, such as naturally fermented sauerkraut, pickled vegetables, fermented grains and fermented juices. According to Dr. Johannes Kuhl, the originator of the lactic acid fermentation diet for cancer, 50 to 75% of the daily diet should be made up of lactic acid fermented foods.[60]

5. A moderate amount of easily-digested proteins must be eaten. These should be mostly of vegetable origin, such as green leafy vegetables, potatoes, sprouted seeds and grains, nuts and **kvark** (raw, unheated, homemade cottage cheese from high quality unpasterized milk).

6. Avoid completely all other animal proteins: no meat, fowl, eggs or fish. Exception: some biological doctors advise the use of raw liver, preferably calf liver from 100% healthy animals, in small amounts.[24, 44, 45] Some other doctors do not use raw liver, but advocate the use of raw egg yokes from fertile eggs.[45]

7. Take no milk or milk products except the aforementioned **kvark** and soured milks, The best forms of soured milks are: bifidus milk, acidophilus milk, natural buttermilk, and homemade soured milk (clabber-milk), perferably made from goat's milk. Goat's milk is better than cow's milk. Raw goat's milk of high quality contains anti-cancer and anti-arthritis factors.

8. Avoid saturated, cholesterol-rich animal fats, including butter. These should be replaced with a moderate use of **genuine**, cold-pressed vegetable oils, especially sunflower seed oil, flaxseed oil, soy bean oil and safflower oil. Oils should never be heated. (Note: most vegetable oils produced in the U.S. **are** heated). If used in cooking, they should be added after the food is cooked. Carcinogenic substances are produced in vegetable oils during prolonged heating.[22]   Dr. Issels says, "It has been established conclusively that avoidance of animal fats, including butter, will diminish the risk of cancer."

9. Eliminate from the diet all processed and denatured foods, especially all refined carbohydrates, such as white flour and white sugar, and all foods made with them.

3. ELIMINATION OF RANCID AND STALE FOODS

All health-conscious people, but particularly those who are cancer-prone and those who already have cancer, should never use rancid or stale foods. As I mentioned before, all rancid foods contain carcinogenic substances.[21]   Dr. H. Anemueller says, "During the oxidation process harmful chemical substances are produced in foods. These substances irritate the delicate lining of the stomach and intestines. Prolonged use of rancid oils or foods can, under some conditions, have a carcinogenic effect — in other words, they can cause cancer ... "

Therefore, an anti-cancer diet should include only 100% fresh foods. All seeds, nuts and grains should be consumed whole, or ground immediately before use. Particular care should be exercised in regard to vegetable oils. Most oils sold in the United States, although advertised and labeled as "cold pressed." actually are not. They are processed by heat and chemical solvent extraction. There is no such thing as cold pressed wheat germ oil, for example. But since there is no law against it, unscrupulous manfacturers label it "cold pressed." Rancid oils can be identified by the characteristic smell and an acrid, throat-burning aftertaste.

4. CLEANSING JUICE FASTING

One of the most important components of the total, combined anti-cancer program is the detoxification of the whole body. The underlying reason why the organism succumbs to cancer in the first place, is the diminished or broken down resistance to the carcinogenic factors mainly due to the disordered metabolism, weakened activity of essential organs, such as liver, kidneys and pancreas, and general auto-toxemia. The purpose of juice fasting is to normalize all the vital body processes, revitalize the liver and other cleansing organs, cleanse the whole body of accumulated toxins, restore the digestive and assimilative functions of the stomach and intestinal tract, and, in general, increase the body's protective and healing capacity. The success of most anti-cancer programs in European biological clinics, as well as the Gerson's cancer therapy, or Dr. Kelley's program, is attributed largely to their thorough cleansing programs. [26, 42, 43, 44]

Short, repeated cleansing fasts on raw vegetable and fruit juices are advisable. Most useful juices are: red beet (from tops and roots), [61] carrot, green juice (made from leafy green vegetables, grape, [62] lemon, and all dark-colored juices. During fasting, daily coffee enemas are used — one cup of strong, freshly brewed coffee in one pint of water, used as a retention enema — to stimulate the liver and increase its detoxifying activity. Although healthy persons can fast on their own, cancer patients should fast only under sympathetic professional supervision.[26, 44, 47]

28

5. SYSTEMATIC UNDEREATING

Systematic overeating, and consequent obesity, is one of the main causes of all disease, including cancer. This was clearly understood many thousands of years ago. In 3,800 B.C. (almost 6,000 years ago!) the following inscription was made in an Egyptian pyramid: "Man lives on ¼ of what he eats. On the other ¾ lives his doctor."

The anti-cancer diet is a prudent diet based on systematic undereating, rather than overeating. Especially in regard to proteins overindulgence is extremely dangerous. Leading cancer researchers agree that overindulgence in proteins and the body's inability to properly utilize them, is one of the main causes of cancer. All overeating, but particularly over-eating of proteins, has a destructive, paralyzing effect on the liver, pancreas and kidneys, those vital organs most involved in the protective mechanism against cancer development.[24]

Unfortunately, not only the average layman, but even the "elect ones", like some of our leading health writers, have been misled by the propaganda and the slanted research paid for by meat and dairy industries. Consequently, through ex-aggerated and unscientific emphasis on the importance of protein, they have helped to create the present high-protein fad in this country. As the inevitable result, while we lead the world in protein consumption, we also lead the world in most degenerative diseases, including cancer.

There is rapidly accumulating evidence from the most reliable research centers of the world, that the high protein fad has no base in scientific fact. Our protein beliefs were based on erroneous calculations of some nineteenth-century scientists such as Rubner, Von Voit and Von Liebig. Recent independent and reliable studies brought forth three revolu-tionary discoveries:

1. That our actual protein need for optimum health is much lower than previously calculated. This is the reason why the official National Research Council re-

commendation for daily protein has been consistently going down, from 120 grams of three decades ago to the present 55 grams. The actual need is even less than that — between 25 and 50 grams a day.[48]

2. That eating more protein than we actually need is extremely dangerous, resulting in autotoxemia and many diseases, including cancer.[24]

3. That many vegetable proteins (especially soybeans, buckwheat, almonds, sesame seeds, sunflower seeds, potatoes, sprouted seeds and grains, and all green vegetables) are biologically superior to meat proteins. Also, raw proteins (which can be more easily obtained from vegetable sources than from meat) are twice as easily digested and utilized as cooked proteins. This means that you can cut your protein intake in half if your protein foods are consumed in the natural, raw state.[48]

A high protein diet is particularly dangerous for older people, whose enzyme and gastric juice production is slowed down. Thus, they cannot digest or utilize proteins effectively. The solution is not overtaxing the digestive, eliminative and cleansing system by eating more proteins and taking hydrochloric acid and other acids, but lowering the protein intake, with emphasis on raw proteins of vegetable origin plus easily-digestible and assimilable proteins of kvark, the homemade, unheated cottage cheese.[24, 48]

It is also extremely important that cancer patients (or those who wish to prevent cancer) eat several small meals a day, rather than a few large ones.

6. ANTI-CANCER SUPPLEMENTS

The following vitamins, minerals, and food supplements have been found to posess anti-cancer properties that help the body's resistance and promote protective and healing activity against cancer:

- **Vitamin A** — large doses up to 150,000 units a day [34, 36, 49, 50] Vitamin A deficiency definitely contributes to the development of cancer.

- **Brewer's yeast** — 3 to 4 tablespoons a day, dry or live yeast.[24]   Yeast is an extremely nutritious, cleansing and cancer-preventative food. (Note: Use only food yeast. Do not use yeast intended for baking.)
- **Vitamin F** — or essential fatty acids (cold-pressed vegetable oils)[24,59]
- **Vitamin B$_{15}$** (pangamic acid) — 100 mg. daily. Many scientists believe that chronic oxygen deficiency in cells leads to the formation of cancer cells (Warburg, Goldblatt, et al.). Vitamin B$_{15}$ increases the body's resistance to oxygen deficiency.[48]
- **Vitamin B$_{17}$** (nitrilosides).[51]   This audience is well aware of the value of nitrilosides in cancer treatment. Although still controversial, nitrilosides certainly should not be omitted when a total cancer-approach, as recommended here, is desired, especially in view of the fact that nitrilosides are completely harmless.[51]   Best food sources of vitamin B$_{17}$, or nitrilosides, are: mung beans, lima beans, lentils, shell beans, crab apples, cranberries, peaches, plums, apricots, cherries and apples (the latter eaten whole, including seeds) Sprouted seeds, particularly sprouted mung beans and lentils, are excellent sources.
- **Vitamin C** — large doses of 5,000 mg. or more a day. Vitamin C is the most potent anti-toxin known. It can effectively neutrilize or minimize the damaging effect of most chemical carcinogens in food and environment — and, thus, be of great value in cancer prevention programs, as well as in the treatment of cancer.[50, 52]
- **Vitamin E** — up to 1,000 I.U. a day. Vitamin C and E can help the body inhibit the activity of the enzyme hyaluronidase, found in cancerous tissue. Vitamin E also increases the oxygenation of cells, which is of crucial importance both in prevention and treatment of cancer.[24, 55]

- **Vitamin B-Complex,** natural, high potency — important for the prevention of cirrhosis of the liver which often leads to cancer. The incidence of cancer in liver that has been affected by cirrhosis is 60 times greater than in normal liver. Also, studies show that B-vitamin deficient diets lead to a higher incidence of primary liver cancer than B-vitamin rich diets.[16, 54, 56]

   Dr. Otto Warburg, Nobel Prize winner and director of the Max Plank Institute for Cell Physiology in Berlin, and one of the leading cancer experts in the world, says that the primary cause of cancer is the lack of one or more of three B-vitamins — riboflavin, niacin and pantothenic acid — in tissues subjected to carcinogens. Dr. Warburg says that a plentiful supply of these three vitamins in the diet is the best possible protection against cancer.[57]

- **Comprehensive mineral and trace element supplement,** particularly rich in potassium.[44, 63] Potassium deficiency is considered by many (Gerson, Scott, etc.) as a main contributing cause of cancer.

- **Comprehensive digestive enzyme supplement,** rich in pancreatic enzymes, to help the body better utilize nutrients, particularly proteins.[26]

7. NON-TOXIC UNORTHODOX THERAPIES

Because the orthodox medicine approves only the three methods by which cancer may be treated — surgery, radiation and chemotherapy — many "unorthodox" therapies for cancer have been developed during the last few decades. Most of these are non-toxic, most have proven to be effective in the control of cancer and/or effecting the betterment of the condition. We list here some of the most popular non-toxic treatments with references for further study.

- Hypotonic therapy [64]
- Glyoxylide, or Kochs treatment[65]
- Hoxsey herbs[66]

- Laetrile[67]
- Krebiozen and Carcalon[68]

A good source of information on these and many other non-toxic cancer treatments is an informative book, **March of Truth on Cancer.**[69] The International Association of Cancer Victims and Friends[70] may help the reader to obtain the available printed material about non-toxic therapies and about qualified doctors who give some of these treatments.

It is our opinion, however, that these therapies, which are mainly aimed at destroying cancer cells and "controlling" cancer, should be used **only** as an adjunct to the **total** anti-cancer program as suggested in this paper. Although some of these treatments may be effective in destroying cancer cells and eliminating the symptoms, they do not eliminate the **underlying causes** which lead to the development of cancer. Only the **total** program of cleansing the body of carcinogenic toxins, strengthening the body's own healing forces by various supportive measures, as described in this book, and eliminating all the carcinogenic factors from man's environment and food, can help the body to cure itself and restore health.

Conclusion:

THE TOTAL APPROACH

It is evident from the above presentation that the basic causes of cancer are known, and have been known for a long time. They are to be found in our denatured environment and health-destroying mode of living: carcinogenic substances in air, soil, water and food; smoking; overindulgence in proteins and the body's inability to properly utilize them; nutritional deficiencies and other physical and emotional stresses which weaken and break down the body's resistance to disease.

It is also evident that the battle against cancer can be won only by massive preventive programs aimed at eliminating all environmental carcinogenic factors, improving our nutritional patterns, and strengthening the body's resistance against disease. When cancer is already manifest, the only program of treatment that will lead to success must be a **total** concerted attack on all fronts aimed at supporting the body's own efforts to heal itself and restore health. The supportive measures, as described in this book, include: artificially induced fever, carcinogen-free diet, internal cleansing program to activate the body's defensive mechanism, special anti-cancer vitamins and other nutritional supplements — all aimed at inhibiting the development of cancer and helping the body to cure itself by its own healing efforts.

Let us keep in mind this concept of totality in our approach to cancer. **Only a total comprehensive preventive and therapeutic anti-cancer approach, a combined, concerted attack on all fronts, as presented in this paper, can assure the needed supportive aid to the body's own protective and healing activity and lead us to a total victory over cancer.**

REFERENCES

1. Rodale, J.I. & Staff, *Cancer — Facts and Fallacies,* Rodale Press, Penna.

2. Corsan, Edward F., Decker, Henry B., Andrews, G.C., et al., as reported to the American Dermatological Association, April 27, 1948.

3. *Encyclopedia of Common Diseases,* Rodale & Staff, Rodale Press, 1970.

4. Homburger F., and Fishman, W.H., *The Physiopathology of Cancer,* Paul B. Hoeber, New York, 1970.

5. Knight, G.F., Martin, Coda W., et al., "Possible Cancer Hazards of Feeding Diethylstilbestrol to Cattle." presented on Congressional Hearings on Food Additives, 1957-58, pp. 283-5.

6. Airola, Paavo O., *Sex and Nutrition,* Award Books, Universal Publishing and Distributing Co., New York, 1970.

7. Turner, James S., *The Chemical Feast,* Grossman Publishers, N.Y., 1970.

8. Hueper, Wilhelm C., Interview, "Lung Cancer: Danger in the Air," *Newsweek,* Jan. 11, 1960.

9. Hueper, W.C., *Information on Environmental Cancer Hazards,* Encyclopedia of Common Dieseases, Rodale Press, 1970.

10. *Bibliography of Cancer Produced by Pure Chemical Compounds,* Oxford University Press.

11. Gershoff, S.N. et al. *Journal of Nutrition,* 73:308, 1961.

12. Lindberg, W.O., *American Journal of Clinical Nutrition,* 6, 1958.

13. Friberg, Lars, Prof., reported at Symposium on Environmental Poisons, Stockholm, Nov. 27, 1971.

14. Taylor, Alfred, *Proceedings of the Society for Experimental Biology and Medicine,* Vol. 119, p. 252, 1965.

15. Greenstein, J.P., *Biochemistry of Cancer,* Academic Press, New York, 1954.

16. Blond, K., *The Liver and Cancer,* John Wright and Sons, Bristol, England, 1960.

17. *Prevention of Chronic Illness,* Harvard University Press, Cambridge, Mass., 1957.

18. *Cancer News Journal,* Vol. 7, No. 3-4, March-April, 1972.

19. Seeger, P.G., German Medical Journal, *Hippokrates,* Vol. 13, 1951.

20. *Tidskrift For Halsa,* No. 2, February, 1972. Stockholm, Sweden.

21. Ariola, Paavo O., "The Health Hazard of Rancid Foods," *Are You Confused?*. Health Plus Publishers, P.O. Box 22001, Phoenix, Arizona, 1971.

22. Ivy, A.C., *Gastroenterology,* March, 1955.

23. *Modern Nutrition,* August, 1953.

24. Issels, Josef, "Nutritional Protection Against Cancer," *Tidskrift För Hälsa,* Numbers 2, 3, and 4, 1972, Stockholm, Sweden.

25. Engel, R.W. et al., *Cancer Research,* 11:180, 1951.

26. Kelley, William Donald, *One Answer to Cancer,* The Kelley Research Foundation, 1971.

27. Sokoloff, Boris, *Cancer, New Approaches, New Hope,* Devin-Adair, New York.

28. *The Challenge of Cancer,* published by the National Cancer Institute.

29. *Nutrition Reviews,* 4:353, 1946.

30. *The American Journal of Pathology,* September, 1946.

31. Voluter, G., et al., *Nutr. Abstract Review,* 30, 975, 1960.

32. Davis, Adelle, *Let's Get Well,* Harcourt, Brace & World, Inc., New York, 1965.

33. Wynder, E.L., et al., *Cancer,* 12, 1959.

34. Kreshover, Seymore, et al., *Journal of the American Dental Association,* April 1957.

35. Voisin, Andre, *Soil, Grass and Cancer* (reference to the research at Winnepeg Hospital, Canada), Philosophical Press.

36. Shamberger, Raymond J., *Journal of National Cancer Institute,* May, 1971.

37. Bois, P., University of Montreal. Report to the Federation of American Societies for Experimental Biology, April, 1968.

38. Lewis, Howard R. and Martha E., *Psychosomatics,* Viking Press, Inc., New York, N.Y.

39. LeShan, Lawrence, *Cancer and Personality: A Critical Review,* Journal of the National Cancer Institute, Jan., 1959.

40. Waerland, Are and Ebba, *Health is Your Birthright,* Humata Publishers, Bern, Switzerland.

41. Lwoff, A., and Lwoff, M., *Ann. Inst. Pasteur,* Sept. 1961.

42. Aly, Karl-Otto, "Cancer Defeated by Body's Own Defenses," *Tidskrift För Hälsa,* Sept., 9, 1965.

43. Airola, Paavo O., *Health Secrets From Europe,* Parker Publishing Co., West Nyack, N.Y., 1970.

44. Gerson, Max, *A Cancer Therapy — Fifty Case Histories,* Dura Books, Inc. 20 Vessey St., New York, N.Y.

45. Unfortunately the liver available in the United States is loaded with carcinogenic toxins and cannot be recommended in the anti-cancer diet. Even the liver of so-called organically raised or wild animals is unfit since they breath contaminated air and drink contaminated water. (The Author)

46. Nolfi, Kristine, *The Raw Food Treatment of Cancer and Other Diseases,* available from Cancer Book House, Solana Beach, California.

47. Airola, Paavo O., *How to Keep Slim, Healthy and Young with Juice Fasting,* Health Plus Publishers, P.O. Box 22001, Phoenix, Arizona, 1971.

48. Airola, Paavo O., *Are You Confused?,* Health Plus Publishers, P.O. Box 22001, Phoenix, Arizona, 1971.

49. "Vitamin A Fights Cancer", *Prevention,* April 1972.

50. Journal of the American Medical Association, August 14, 1954.

51. Krebs, Ernst T., Jr.,   The Nitrilosides (vitamin B-17), *Cancer News Journal,* Vol. 6, 1-4, Jan-April, 1971.

52. Larson, Gena, "Is There An Anti-cancer Food.," *Prevention,* April, 1972.

53. McCormick, W.J., *Archives of Pediatrics,* October, 1954.

54. Krebs, Ernst T., Jr. "Laetrile and Anti-cancer Factors in Our Foods," *Cancer News Journal,* Vol. 5, No. 5-8, May-August, 1970.

55. Adamstone, F.B., *American Journal on Cancer,* 28, 540, 1936.

56. Briggs, N.H., *Australian Journal of Biological Sciences,* 13, 1960.

57. Warburg, Otto.,"Concerning the Ultimate Cause and the Contributing Causes of Cancer," address delivered at a meeting of Nobel Prize Winners in Lindau, Germany, July, 1966.

58. The address for Dr. Josef Issels' clinic in Germany is: Ringberg Klinik, 8183 Rottach-Egern/OBB., Ringbergstrasse 30, West Germany (Phone: 08022-6458 or 6459).

59. Aviles, Humberto, *"Discovery of the Anti-cancerous Properties of Vitamin F",* 2023 West Wisconsin Ave., Milwaukee, Wisc. 53201.

60. Kuhl, Johannes, *"Check Mate for Cancer",* Viadrina Vertag, A. Trowitzch, Braunlage, Harzburger Str. 6, West Germany.

61. Red Beet Juice therapy for cancer and leukemia, as recommended by Dr. Siegmund Schmidt and Dr. A. Ferenezi — *March of Truth on Cancer,* Arlin Brown Inf. Center, P.O. Box 251, Fort Belvoir, Virginia, 22060.

62. "Modified Grape Cure" and "Grape Cure". Information may be obtained from the Arlin Brown Information Center — see address ref. No. 61.

63. Scott, Cyril, *"Victory Over Cancer",* True Health Publishing Co., London, England, According to Scott, the best forms of potassium supplement for treatment of cancer are: potassium bicarbonate and potassium phosphate. Crude black molasses is recommended as a potassium source.

64. Stephens, John T., (Discoverer of Hypotonic Therapy) 1644 21st St., N.W. Washington D.C., 20009.

65. Koch, William, F., M.D., *"The Survival Factor in Neoplastic and Viral Diseases",* available from IACVF, 155-D, S. Highway 101, Solana Beach, Calif. 92075.

66. Information on Hoxsey treatment is given in the book, *March of Truth on Cancer,* Arlin J. Brown Inf. Center, P.O. Box 251, Fort Belvoir, Virginia, 22060.

67. Kittler, Glenn D., *"Laetrile: Control for Cancer".* Paperback Library, 260 Park Ave. S., New York, N.Y. 10000.

68. The Ivy Cancer Research Foundation, 622 West Diversey Parkway, Chicago, Ill. 60614.

69. *March of Truth on Cancer,* The Arlin J. Brown Information Center, P.O. Box 251, Fort Belvoir, Virginia, 22060.

70. The International Association of Cancer Victims and Friends, Inc. Box 707, Solana Beach, Calif. 92075.

RECOMMENDED DAILY

(Designed for the maintenance of good nutrition

BASED ON TABLES PUBLISHED BY FOOD AND NUTRITION
RESEARCH COUNCIL.

	AGE From up to years	WEIGHT kg.	WEIGHT lb.	HEIGHT cm.	HEIGHT in.	ENERGY CALORIES KCAL	PROTEIN GM	VITAMIN A ACTIVITY I.U.	VITAMIN D I.U.	VITAMIN E ACTIVITY I.U.
INFANTS	0.0-0.5	6	14	60	24	kg. x 117	kg. x 2.2	1,400	400	4
	0.5-1.0	9	20	71	28	kg. x 108	kg. x 2.0	2,000	400	5
CHILDREN	1-3	13	28	86	34	1,300	23	2,000	400	7
	4-6	20	44	110	44	1,800	30	2,500	400	9
	7-10	30	66	135	54	2,400	36	3,300	400	10
MALES	11-14	44	97	158	63	2,800	44	5,000	400	12
	15-18	61	134	172	69	3,000	54	5,000	400	15
	19-22	67	147	172	69	3,000	52	5,000	400	15
	23-50	70	154	172	69	2,700	56	5,000	—	15
	51+	70	154	172	69	2,400	56	5,000	—	15
FEMALES	11-14	44	97	155	62	2,400	44	4,000	400	10
	15-18	54	119	162	65	2,100	48	4,000	400	11
	19-22	58	128	162	65	2,100	46	4,000	400	12
	23-50	58	128	162	65	2,000	46	4,000	—	12
	51+	58	128	162	65	1,800	46	4,000	—	12
	Pregnant					+300	+30	5,000	400	15
	Lactating					+500	+20	6,000	400	15

FAT-SOLUBLE VITAMINS (spans VITAMIN A ACTIVITY, VITAMIN D, VITAMIN E ACTIVITY)

DIETARY ALLOWANCES

of practically all healthy people in the U.S.A.)

BOARD, NATIONAL ACADEMY OF SCIENCE, NATIONAL
Revised 1973

WATER-SOLUBLE VITAMINS							MINERALS					
VITAMIN C	FOLACIN	NIACIN	B_2	B_1	B_6	B_{12}	CALCIUM	PHOSPHORUS	IODINE	IRON	MAGNESIUM	ZINC
mg	mcg.	mg.	mg.	mg.	mg.	mcg.	mg.	mg.	mcg.	mg.	mg.	mg.
35	50	5	0.4	0.3	0.3	0.3	360	240	35	10	60	3
35	50	8	0.6	0.5	0.4	0.3	540	400	45	15	70	5
40	100	9	0.8	0.7	0.6	1.0	800	800	60	15	150	10
40	200	12	1.1	0.9	0.9	1.5	800	800	80	10	200	10
40	300	16	1.2	1.2	1.2	2.0	800	800	100	10	250	10
45	400	18	1.5	1.4	1.6	3.0	1,200	1,200	130	18	350	15
45	400	20	1.8	1.5	1.8	3.0	1,200	1,200	150	18	400	15
45	400	20	1.8	1.5	2.0	3.0	800	800	140	10	350	15
45	400	18	1.6	1.4	2.0	3.0	800	800	130	10	350	15
45	400	16	1.5	1.2	2.0	3.0	800	800	110	10	350	15
45	400	16	1.3	1.2	1.6	3.0	1,200	1,200	115	18	300	15
45	400	14	1.4	1.1	2.0	3.0	1,200	1,200	115	18	300	15
45	400	14	1.4	1.1	2.0	3.0	800	800	100	18	300	15
45	400	13	1.2	1.0	2.0	3.0	800	800	100	18	300	15
45	400	12	1.1	1.0	2.0	3.0	800	800	80	10	300	15
60	800	+2	+0.3	+0.3	2.5	4.0	1,200	1,200	125	18+	450	20
60	600	+4	+0.5	+0.3	2.5	4.0	1,200	1,200	150	18	450	25

PAAVO AIROLA'S BOOKS

"I wish to compliment you on your brilliant and dynamic presentation of contemporary health problems and how they can be overcome in a most logical and convincing sequence. I have received great pleasure and stimulation from reading your books, and feel you have given to the Western world some priceless teachings which they are so pathetically in need of."

Dr. M.O. Garten, N.D., D.C., San Jose, California

"I have recently purchased your book, HOW TO GET WELL. I want to commend you for a very excellent book which will be a valuable guide in any physician's office."

Dr. David R. Anderson, M.A., N.D.
Wheeling, Illinois

"I feel that your fasting book is a masterpiece. I have fasted many times in the past on water, but your juice-fasting method is superior — I am on my 28th day of juice fast now."

F. C. Winters, Phoenix, Arizona

"Your book, HOW TO GET WELL, is wonderful . . . Congratulations that the first edition sold out so soon! This do-it-yourself sort of book is what the public is hungry for. No one deserves more than yourself the success you are having — you have worked hard many years and HAVE LIVED BY YOUR PHILOSOPHY as a dynamic example of what you teach."

Betty Lee Morales, Nutrition Consultant,
President, Cancer Control Society,
Secretary, National Health Federation

"Dr. Airola is not only the most knowledgeable, but also the most honest writer of them all."

Dr. Kathlene M. Fricia, D.C., Pasadena, California

"Dr. Paavo Airola has done it again. This time it's HOW TO GET WELL — the crowning glory of his 30 years of the most discriminating world-wide research. With this book he firmly established the fact which we, a few of his long-time followers, knew all along — that he is THE MOST OUTSTANDING NUTRITIONIST in the world today."

Richard Barmakian, Nutrition Consultant,
Pasadena, California

"Please send me a copy of Paavo Airola's HOW TO GET WELL. I am considering one or two of his books emphasizing biological medicine as text books in my Honors Class on nutrition-health relationship. I know of no better author on such matters."

Dr. Louis Junker, Professor of Economics
Western Michigan University

"I am an M.D. with an open mind. I am employing your programs, described in "There Is A Cure For Arthritis", and they are actually doing wonders for my patients."

Dr. T., M.D., Grafton, W. Virginia

"Thank you so much for the recent book order. Airola's book, HOW TO GET WELL, is a superior book to all that I have read on the subject of getting well."

John Mastel, Health Food Store Owner,
St. Paul, Minnesota

"In all sincerity. I find that your books, particularly "Health Secrets From Europe" and "There Is A Cure For Arthritis", are my very best references on the many aspects of health, and they have been most helpful to me and my practice of any that I have gotten — and I have an extensive library. I find that "Are You Confused?" has straightened out a lot of questions in my mind."

Dr. E. W. Conroy, Kaitaia, New Zealand

"I find your book, "Are You Confused?", excellent in every way . . . I believe the last chapter, Biological Medicine, is worth the price of the book alone."

Dr. C. Serritella, D.C., Caribou, Maine

"Your book, HOW TO GET WELL, is sensational! I am impressed with the way in which you conceived and constructed it, with your fabulous and expert presentation of the philosophy of biological medicine, and with common and academic sense that it makes . . . There are but few informed and courageous leaders concerned with the well-being of the public; leaders who have not only dedicated their lives to helping their fellow men, but who have the sufficient knowledge and qualifications to accomplish this. I am proud to tell you that I feel you to be one of those few. By writing this book, you rendered a great service to a disease-ridden mankind."

Dr. H. Rudolph Alsleben, M.D., Anaheim, California

"No doubt in my mind about it — you are the Number One nutritionist and the most knowledgeable health writer."

Audry Smith, Reg. Therapist. Escondido, California

"Congratulations on your fabulous new book. HOW TO GET WELL is doubtlessly the book of the century! At our store, it is selling better than even our paperbacks!"

Scott S. Smith, Vegetarian World.

"We think your book, "Are You Confused" is a masterpiece. It should be a must reading for everyone who wants to get a good idea on how to achieve real health."

Robert Yaller, Santa Monica, California

"Paavo Airola's book, HOW TO GET WELL, is interesting, informative, and helpful. $8.95 worth of information on every page!"

I. M. Marynak, Skokie, Illinois

"Are You Confused?" is our bible."

Mr. J. H. B., San Francisco, California

"I stayed up all night reading your book . . . It's terrific."

Rev. Robert Strecker, Los Angeles, California

"I am congratulating you for your pioneer work. Your work will contribute to the freedom of thought and of therapeutic alternatives — and, thus, to the improvement of the health standards in your country."

Dr. Lars-Erik Essén, M.D., Sweden

"HOW TO GET WELL is a tremendous book and it sells itself. Our customers agree that it is the most popular and informative book we have stocked at any time. We feel that it is 1974's best seller in the health book field."

Carl P. Pearson, Health Food Store Owner, Mount Vernon, Washington

(There are hundreds of similar unsolicited comments in publishers' files.)

ABOUT THE AUTHOR

Paavo Airola, Ph.D., N.D., is an internationally-recognized nutritionist, naturopathic physician, educator, and award-winning author. Raised and educated in Europe, he studied biochemistry, nutrition, and natural healing in biological medical centers of Sweden, Germany, and Switzerland. He lectures extensively world-wide, both to professionals and laymen, holding yearly educational seminars for physicians. He has been a visiting lecturer at many universities and medical schools, including the Stanford University Medical School.

Dr. Paavo Airola is the author of thirteen widely-read books, notably his two international best-sellers, *How To Get Well,* and *Are You Confused?* The American Academy of Public Affairs issued Dr. Airola the Award of Merit for his book on arthritis.

How To Get Well, the comprehensive Handbook of Natural Healing, is the most authoritative and practical manual on biological medicine in print. It is used as a textbook in several universities and medical schools, and regarded as a reliable reference manual, the "Bible of Natural Healing," by doctors, researchers, nutritionists, and students of health and holistic healing. Dr. Airola's book, *Hypoglycemia: A Better Approach,* has revolutionized the therapeutic concept of this insidious, complex, and devastating affliction.

Dr. Airola's newest monumental work, *Everywoman's Book,* is a great new contribution in the field of holistic medicine. It not only confirms Dr. Airola's unchallenged leadership in the field of nutrition and holistic healing, but demonstrates his genius as an original thinker, philosopher, and profound humanitarian.

Dr. Airola is President of the International Academy of Biological Medicine; a member of the International Naturopathic Association; and a member of the International Society for Research on Civilization Diseases and Environment, the prestigious Forum for world-wide research founded by Dr. Albert Schweitzer. Dr. Airola is listed in the *Directory of International Biography,* in *The Blue Book, The Men of Achievement, Who's Who in American Art,* and *Who's Who in the West.*

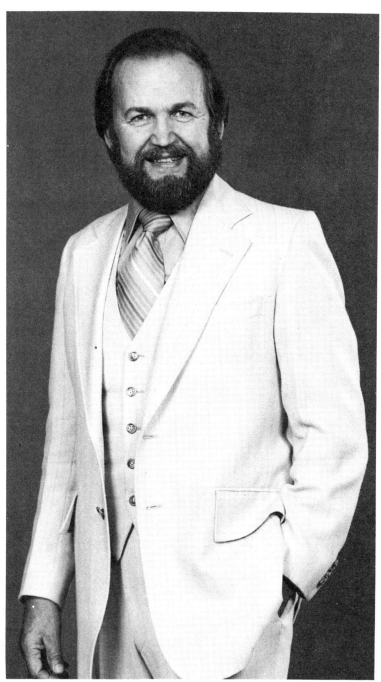
Photo by Diane Padys

NOTES

NOTES

NOTES

NOTES

NOTES